Heal your teeth

Relationship of
physical to dental ailment

Dr. Wolfgang Kuhl

Heal your teeth

Relationship of
physical to dental ailment

Bibliografische Information der Deutschen Nationalbibliothek:
Die Deutsche Nationalbibliothek verzeichnet diese Publikation
in der Deutschen Nationalbibliografie;
detaillierte bibliografische Daten sind im Internet über
http://dnb.d-nb.de abrufbar.

© 2009 Dr. Wolfgang Kuhl
Layout, cover, printing and production:
Books on Demand GmbH, Norderstedt

ISBN: 978-3-8370-2376-3

For Joanna

Content

1. Preface

When I started to work as a dentist in 1989, I thought my responsibility would be to keep teeth healthy and make them more beautiful. Keeping 28 (32) teeth plus 20 milk teeth in good condition seemed to be easy and clear. All my experience since then has led me to the conclusion that nature always does things better than us. A naturally healthy tooth is the best and most durable chewing apparatus that exists. And yet I quite often faced dental problems that could not be explained with limited dentistry thinking. These problems impelled me to further research.

There were some teeth that simply could not be saved or corrected despite all the dentist's knowledge and artful experience. Adjacent teeth were completely intact while the relevant tooth was totally destroyed. There was only one explanation: Other physical and psychological influences were impacting the condition of our teeth. I noticed quite often that people with healthy teeth were healthy in all other aspects as well: this was a first step to viewing teeth from a more psychosomatic perspective.

One essential conclusion is that maintaining and taking good care of our teeth provides the basis for a holistic sense of health and well-being. In other words, it is quite interesting to pose the question, which physical and psychological influences can have a negative impact on our teeth. This book tries to answer that question.

My aim is to provide a multitude of readers a simple and understandable booklet from which they derive great benefits. Furthermore I would like to achieve that, by reading my book, potential other health problems may be recognized and treated at an earlier stage.

If you should like to offer new ideas or criticism, please write an email to info@drkuhl.de. I am looking forward to hear from you and hope you enjoy reading this unusual booklet.

Dr. Wolfgang Kuhl,
February 2009

2. Tooth diagram

An adult normally has 32 permanent teeth. Of these, four are incisors (numbers 1 and 2) and two are canine teeth (number 3) respectively located in the upper and the lower jaw.

Furthermore there are the premolars (numbers 4 and 5) and the molars (numbers 6 and 7), two each on each side of the jaw. The last molar (number 8) is the wisdom tooth. There can be one of them on each side of the upper and lower gums.

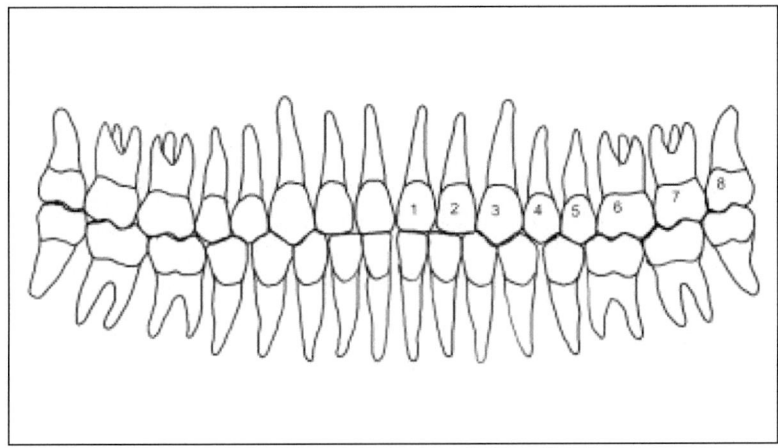

Tooth diagram

3. Symptoms Description

Directions for using the following table:

The first column contains the name of an ailment or a symptom. The second column indicates which teeth can cause the problem described in the first column. These teeth may have caries, fillings, root canal treatments, caps or other kinds of dental substitutes. The third column lists either a description of the cause or other organs that may be related to the problem and that should be checked as well.

Ailment/ Symptoms	Problem teeth	Cause/Effect
Abnormal fatigue / tiredness	All teeth with caps or fillings	Incompatible materials used in caps, fillings and implants (be wary of special offers, discounted service and products from foreign sources). Frequently used metals such as mercury, palladium and tin can easily be detected via urine analysis.
Acne	All incisors	Bladder, kidneys, sexual organs, build-up of toxins and hormonal problems

Ailment/ Symptoms	Problem teeth	Cause/Effect
Adrenal gland	Lower incisors, left and right	Bladder, kidneys, sexual organs
Allergy	Lower incisors, left and right	Incompatibility of materials used for caps, fillings, implants as well as metals, plastics, cements and amalgam that can cause an allergic reaction, if combined with a low physical adaptation to these materials. Bladder, kidneys
Alzheimer disease	All affected teeth	Toxins from non-vital teeth as well as residual amalgam in the tissue are also considered to be contributing causes of Alzheimer's.
Anal itching	All premolars	Colon, lung, maxillary sinus
Anterior pituitary	Upper wisdom teeth	Small intestine
Arteries	Lower molars, left and right	Pancreas, spleen, stomach

Ailment/ Symptoms	Problem teeth	Cause/Effect
Arteriosclerosis	Lower incisors, left and right	Bladder, kidneys, sexual organs
Bladder ailment	All incisors	Brain, kidneys, back of the knee, lumbar spine, sexual organs (male and female), frontal sinus. If there are problems with the bladder, it has to be carefully determined whether the root of the affected tooth has to be treated or whether the resection of the top of the root can be helpful.
Brain	All upper incisors, left and right	Bladder, frontal sinus, kidneys, lumbar spine
Breathing problems	All premolars	Colon, maxillary sinus
Bronchial asthma	All premolars	Colon, maxillary sinus
Bronchitis	All premolars	Colon, maxillary sinus

Ailment/ Symptoms	Problem teeth	Cause/Effect
Burning sensation of the gums	All affected teeth	Black fillings caused by the spread of metal-ions (battery effect)
Burning tongue (glossalgia)	All affected teeth	Black fillings caused by spreading of metal-ions (battery effect)
Central nervous system	Upper wisdom teeth, left and right	Heart, small intestine
Cervical spine	All premolars	Colon, maxillary sinus, lungs
Chest pain, left side	Lower right molars	Pancreas, spleen, stomach
Chest pain, right side	Lower left molars	Pancreas, spleen, stomach
Chewing gum	All molars and premolars	Chewing gum confuses the digestive system. Digestive juices are constantly made available but not utilized. Constant chewing of gum is harmful to the jaw if there is a pre-existing damage.

Ailment/ Symptoms	Problem teeth	Cause/Effect
Chronic fatigue syndrome	All teeth with caps or fillings	Incompatible materials used in caps, fillings or implants (be wary of special offers, discounted service and products from foreign sources). Frequently-used metals such as mercury, palladium and tin can easily be detected via urine analysis.
Colitis (inflammation of the colon)	All premolars	Lung, maxillary sinus
Colon disorders (constipation, diarrhea)	All premolars	Lung, maxillary sinus
Contact problems with other people	All affected teeth	Bad breath, reserved behavior because of ugly, neglected or missing teeth respectively inharmonious incisors. If a person has poorly done front caps or badly fitting artificial teeth or dentures, speaking problems may occur. This can be a very embarrassing condition.

Ailment/ Symptoms	Problem teeth	Cause/Effect
Deafness	All incisors and wisdom teeth	Heart, small intestine
Debilitating circulation	All wisdom teeth	Ear, small intestine
Depression, external reason	All visible teeth (front teeth)	Ugly, dark and twisted teeth have a negative impact on a person's disposition. People smile very restrainedly or suppress smiling altogether. Having a negative self-image makes one sad, unhappy and in the long run depressive.
Depression, internal reason	Molars and premolars, wisdom teeth	People who have no side teeth or have completely lost their teeth are not able to work on their problems during the night by grinding their teeth. Tooth grinding has the positive effect of generating a huge amount of anti-stress hormones. If these hormones are not regularly generated, it will lead to fatigue and burn-out.

Ailment/ Symptoms	Problem teeth	Cause/Effect
Diabetes	All premolars	Spleen, stomach. In case of advanced periodontitis, organisms from the spleen and their toxins penetrate the circulatory system and can trigger diabetes.
Diarrhea	All premolars	Lungs, maxillary sinus
Dizziness (vertigo)	All wisdom teeth	Heart, small intestine
Earache	All wisdom teeth	Heart, small intestine
Eczema	All incisors	Bladder, kidneys, sexual organs
Elbow	All wisdom teeth	Ear, heart, small intestine
Energy level of the teeth, general	All wisdom teeth	The wisdom teeth are situated in the heart circulation meridian. The latter has to be paid special attention to, in case of constantly low energy level.

Ailment/ Symptoms	Problem teeth	Cause/Effect
Enuresis	All incisors	Kidneys, sexual organs
Eye ailment	All canine teeth	Gallbladder, hip, liver, thoracic spine
Eye, left and right	Incisors left and right upper jaw	Gallbladder; hip, liver, posterior pituitary, thoracic spine
Fatigue, chronic	Lower wisdom teeth, left and right	Bladder, kidneys (poor elimination of toxins results in fatigue); exclude suspicion of tumor.
Frequent urinating	All incisors	Kidneys, prostate gland, sexual organs
Frontal sinus	All incisors	Bladder, brain, kidneys
Furuncle (boil)	All incisors	Bladder, kidneys, reduced elimination of toxins, sexual organs

Ailment/ Symptoms	Problem teeth	Cause/Effect
Gallbladder	All canine teeth	Eye, hip, gonads, back of the knee, liver, posterior pituitary, thoracic spine. If problems with the gallbladder exist, the dentist has to examine carefully whether the canine teeth are appropriate anchors for artificial teeth.
Gas problems/ flatulence	All wisdom teeth	Ear, heart
Gastritis	All molars	Pancreas, spleen
Gonads	Second incisor, canine tooth, premolars right lower jaw	Colon, gallbladder, liver
Gum problems	All affected teeth	Inadequate ability to chew. Chewing is good exercise for gum and teeth.

Ailment/ Symptoms	Problem teeth	Cause/Effect
Gum problems, psychological	All affected teeth	Normally there is a balance between bacteria in the mouth and gums and the immune system. In phases of increased stress the defense of the immune system is disturbed, which leads to a malfunction: The body is overtaxed. A major cause for tissue damage is due to the immune reaction. Stress related tooth-grinding puts more strain on the teeth across the axis, similar to the movements of a forceps pulling a tooth. In this way gum and dental attachments are clearly more stressed. Strain on the chewing-musculature, neck and nape pain, tenseness in the head.

Ailment/ Symptoms	Problem teeth	Cause/Effect
Halitosis	All affected teeth	Putrefaction caused by food particles left between the teeth, insufficiently cleaned dentures, caries, poor fillings or caps and bacterial coverage of the tongue. Unfavorably positioned teeth make cleaning and brushing difficult. Personal contact may become problematic.
Hearing, middle ear	All wisdom teeth	Heart, small intestine
Heart	All wisdom teeth	Ear, small intestine
Heart attack, symptoms	All wisdom teeth	A painful wisdom tooth without diagnosis can be an indicator of a heart attack.
Heart disease	All wisdom teeth, general inflammation of the gum	Bacteria and their toxins can adhere to cardiac valves and cause damage.
Heartburn	All molars	Pancreas, spleen, stomach

Ailment/ Symptoms	Problem teeth	Cause/Effect
Hemorrhoids	All premolars	Colon, maxillary sinus, lungs
Hepatitis	All canine teeth	Eye, gallbladder, hip
Hip	All canine teeth	Eye, back of the knee, gallbladder, gonads, liver, posterior pituitary. Disorder of bite with deviation of the lower jar to one side, spine problems
Hoarseness	All premolars	Colon, lung
Hypertension	All wisdom teeth	Small intestine
Immune deficiency	All molars	Pancreas, spleen, stomach
Immune system	All molars	Pancreas, spleen, stomach
Impotence	All incisors	Bladder, kidneys. The incisors relate directly to the male sexual organs and their hormonal control. Non-vital incisors can have an intense negative impact on male virility.

Ailment/ Symptoms	Problem teeth	Cause/Effect
Indigestion	All second molars and premolars	Compare stomach problems. Proper chewing is not possible, so that food is not properly crushed and blended with saliva and digestive enzymes. Food reaches the stomach without adequate preparation. The consequence is that nutrients are poorly utilized.
Inflammation of the middle ear	All wisdom teeth	Heart, small intestine
Inflammation of the mucous membrane	All molars	Pancreas, spleen, stomach
Irritated throat	All molars	If a person grinds their teeth very often, the lower tongue muscles get shorter. This phenomenon stimulates coughing by leading to a constant tension on the bronchia.
Jaundice	All canine teeth	Eye, gallbladder, hip

Ailment/ Symptoms	Problem teeth	Cause/Effect
Kidney discomfort	All incisors	Bladder, sexual organs. In case of kidney problems, it has to be carefully determined, whether a root canal treatment on the affected tooth or the resection of the top of the root can be therapeutically effective.
Knee	All incisors and canine teeth	Bladder, kidneys, liver, spine
Larynx	Premolars left lower jaw	Colon, lungs
Legs of different length	All molars and premolars	Bite disorder with deviation of the lower jaw to one side. Spine problems due to attempts to compensate for the deviation.

Ailment/ Symptoms	Problem teeth	Cause/Effect
Liver	All canine teeth	Eye, gallbladder, gonads, hip, posterior pituitary, thoracic spine. In case of an existing liver ailment, the dentist has to check carefully whether the canine teeth are appropriate anchors for prostheses.
Lumbar spine	All middle incisors	Bladder, brain, kidneys
Lung	All premolars	Colon, maxillary sinus
Lymphatic vessels	Lower second molar, left and right	Pancreas, spleen, stomach

Ailment/ Symptoms	Problem teeth	Cause/Effect
Malnutrition	Absence of all affected teeth	Inadequate chewing ability because of bad or missing teeth as well as poorly fitting dentures leads people to select their food according to the motto"Is it easy to chew?" Food choices and variety are clearly limited. Temporary alternatives are liquid nourishment. In general, this results in diminished body function and overall weakness. There is no enjoyment in eating.
Maxillary sinus	All premolars	Colon, lungs
Menopause discomforts	All incisors	Bladder, kidneys, sexual organs
Menstruation problems	All incisors	Bladder, kidneys, sexual organs
Metallic taste in the mouth	All teeth with caps or fillings	Oxidation processes and battery effect due to different metals in the mouth
Miscarriage	All incisors	Bladder, kidneys

Ailment/ Symptoms	Problem teeth	Cause/Effect
Nasal sinus cavity	All premolars	Colon, lungs
Neck problems	All molars, premolars and wisdom teeth (teeth grinding and pressing at night)	Abnormal biting or grinding with a pressure of 300 to 400 kilograms leads to muscle tension in the cervical muscle and in the neck.
Nose breathing, limited	Missing premolars	If the premolars in the upper jaw are pulled too early, this can lead to a poorly developed nose area. This will cause a less effective capability of breathing through the nose.
Oropharynx	All molars	Pancreas, spleen, stomach
Pancreas	All molars	Spleen, stomach
Pancreatitis	Lower and upper molars, right	Mucous membranes, spleen, stomach
Parathyroid	Upper molars, left and right	Pancreas, stomach

Ailment/ Symptoms	Problem teeth	Cause/Effect
Periodontosis	All affected teeth	Disturbed bacterial balance in the mouth has a negative impact on the intestine. 80 % of the immune system is located in the intestine.
Pneumonia	All premolars	Colon, maxillary sinus
Posterior pituitary	Upper second incisors and canine teeth	Eye, gallbladder, hip, liver (right side), thoracic spine
Pregnancy problems	All incisors	Bladder, kidneys
Pregnancy, effects on teeth	All teeth	The nourishing of the embryo (fetus) draws a huge amount of important vitamins and minerals from the mother's body, so that the supply mineral-rich saliva to the teeth is reduced. Moreover the hormonal adjustment tends to increase the likeliness of a gum inflammation. Pregnancies in close succession are particularly burdensome to the female body.

Ailment/ Symptoms	Problem teeth	Cause/Effect
Premature birth	All affected teeth	In case of periodontosis pathogenic bacteria dismiss carriers which trigger an immune reaction. This can lead to contractions (labor pains) and cause a premature birth.
Psyche	All affected teeth	If a person misses the sweetness of life, it is often replaced with chocolate. It is not without reason that we speak of chocolate as nutrition for the nerves. If, in this case, mouth hygiene is not perfect, decalcification will lead to caries development.
School begin	First molar	If the first molar is not yet visible, perhaps the child is too young to go to school and possibly not sufficiently developed to be ready for school.
Scoliosis / pelvis	All molars and premolars	Disorder of the bite with deviation of the lower jaw to one side

Ailment/ Symptoms	Problem teeth	Cause/Effect
Shoulder	All wisdom teeth	Pain dragging into the shoulder may be an indication of heart problems.
Skin diseases	All incisors	Bladder, kidneys, sexual organs
Skin rash	All affected teeth	Incompatible materials of caps, fillings, implants as well as metals, plastics, cements, amalgam can cause an allergic reaction, if combined with a low physical adaptation to these materials.
Small intestine	All wisdom teeth	Ear, heart
Snoring	Retrusive position of the lower jaw	With increasing age the chewing muscle gets weaker causing the lower jaw to fall backwards and the tongue to narrow the air-way while sleeping. Using a snoring splint might help, because this device stabilizes the lower jaw in a protrusive position to keep the air-way open.

Ailment/ Symptoms	Problem teeth	Cause/Effect
Sphenoid sinus	All incisors	Eye, gallbladder, liver
Spleen	All lower and upper left molars	Stomach
Sterility	All incisors	Sensitivity and vitality of the teeth has to be checked.
Stomach ache/ problems	a) All molars b) All affected teeth	a) Colon, immune system, knee, maxillary sinus, pancreas b) Proper chewing is not possible because of poor artificial teeth, missing or loose and painful teeth.

Ailment/ Symptoms	Problem teeth	Cause/Effect
Taste, no sense of	All affected teeth	a) Black fillings as result of spreading metal-ions b) Artificial teeth (dentures) cover large parts of the mucous membrane, which is responsible for tasting. c) If the sinus cavities are heavily inflamed, the mucous membrane swells on the nerve, inhibiting the ability to smell and taste. The nerve becomes partially numb. It is important to check whether a tumor may be the reason.
Thoracic spine	All second incisors and canine teeth	Eye, gallbladder, gonads, hip, knee, liver, posterior pituitary
Throat ache	All premolars	Colon, lungs
Thyroid gland	Upper incisors, left and right	Bladder, kidneys, sexual organs

Ailment/ Symptoms	Problem teeth	Cause/Effect
Tinnitus	Molars and premolars at the side	Tinnitus is increased by tooth grinding during the night. In the case of an abnormal occlusion, a temporary retainer (brace) is recommended to relieve the condition.
Tonsillitis	All molars	Pancreas, spleen, stomach
Toxication symptoms	Teeth with fillings and root fillings	Toxins from non-vital teeth are among the strongest known.
Urogenital system	All incisors	Bladder, kidneys

Ailment/ Symptoms	Problem teeth	Cause/Effect
Vitamin deficiency	All molars and premolars	Inadequate chewing ability because of bad or missing teeth as well as improperly fitting dentures leads people to select food according to the motto"Is it easy to chew?" Food choices and variety are clearly limited. Temporary alternatives are liquid nourishment. In general, this results in diminished body function and overall weakness. There is no enjoyment in eating.
Wound healing, insufficient, painful	All affected teeth and jaw	Blockage of the upper cervical vertebra may lead to light numbness in face and jaw. Therefore these parts will not be supported with blood properly. If a tooth was extracted the healing of the wound may be disturbed, retarded and moreover very painful.

4. Psychological aspects

Teeth	Meaning
All incisors	They represent the ego and the personal life energy.
All upper incisors	They express female and male eroticism and desirability.
Diastema (gap between middle incisors)	The person has problems integrating his female and male side. The male feels both attracted and rejected by a woman. The female is constantly challenging the man she is living with. The diastema indicates a person's detachment from his parents.
Overlapping of incisors	The protruding tooth indicates the dominant parent.
Upper right middle incisor in front of upper left middle incisor	The paternal influence is dominant in the upbringing of the child.
Upper left middle incisor in front of upper right middle incisor	The maternal part is dominant in the upbringing of the child.

Teeth	Meaning
Trauma and injury to upper right middle incisor	Women have difficulties to prevail in their relationship with the father, husband or partner.
Trauma and injury to upper left middle incisor	Men have difficulties to prevail in their relationship with their mother, wife or partner.
Small incisors on both sides	They indicate a friendly and peaceful character.
Completely nested incisors	Female and male sides are barely developed.
Upper right middle incisor	Represents the male parts within us according to how we relate to the father.
Upper left middle incisor	Represents our female parts according to how we relate to the mother.
Upper left and right middle incisors	They represent basic human energy, as well as nidation (the nesting of the egg in the cell). An emotionally repressed abortion leads to loose incisors in a woman.

Teeth	Meaning
Upper second incisors	Reflect a child's relationship to its parents. If the second incisors grow forward, the child dominates the parents. If they grow backwards, the parents dominate the child. If only one incisor grows backwards or forward, the relationship to either the mother (left) or to the father (right) is affected.
Carious incisors despite dental care	Can be considered as an indication of an emotional problem. If the second incisors on the left side are carious, a man is emotionally disappointed by a woman. If the second incisors on the right side are carious, it is the other way round.

Teeth	Meaning
All canine teeth	They start growing with the onset of puberty. They appear as soon as sexual interest and sexual maturity are developing. Canine teeth are very important for vitality. Disease or problems with canine teeth in the lower jaw quite often diminish vitality dramatically. If problems exist with the liver and gallbladder meridian, canine teeth should better not be used as anchors for artificial teeth.
Missing or delayed break-through of a canine tooth	The person does not take responsibility for his life. Frequently he is a pampered only child.
Upper canine tooth behind lower canine tooth	A male is inhibited from living-out his gender.
Upper right canine tooth	Stands for the way we want to present ourselves to the world.
Upper left canine tooth	Stands for our mental attitude towards changes.

Teeth	Meaning
Lower right canine tooth	Expresses what we want to achieve in the world. At the time of its breakthrough it utilizes all the growth energy. After its breakthrough a physical growth spurt can be noticed.
Lower left canine tooth	Expresses how we display inner changes to the world. With persons, who constantly avoid conflicts, the canine tooth turns and acts evasively.
Upper right second premolar	This premolar shows our worldly development, i.e. children we wish to have, or plans, we would have liked to realize. In women who experience problems in getting pregnant due to infertility, miscarriage or abortion, the premolar is quite often non-vitalized. In a well-functioning relationship the male partner frequently shares the tooth problem.

Teeth	Meaning
Upper left second premolar	This premolar is a special tooth with a karmic meaning. It shows whether we are developing our personality according to our capabilities and whether we are using our hidden abilities. If we obstruct our own way to full development, the premolar will reveal this with tooth problems.
Lower left second premolar	Indicates how we integrate the essence of our mother's nature in our own. If this premolar grows into the inner mouth, we are dealing with an oppressive mother. Self-assertion may be difficult in conflict situations. In conjunction with this, shoulder disorders occur which do not respond to treatment or therapy.
Lower right second premolar	Represents the realization of our plans, especially in the occupational context. Decisive work-related changes could have an effect bearing on this premolar.

Teeth	Meaning
Upper right first molar	Stands for the worldly status we want to have. It gets carious, if some of our plans have not succeeded or resulted in the desired outcome. Pulling the tooth often solves the specific problems.
Upper left first molar	Represents the role we should like to play in order to express our feelings. Caries on this tooth indicates that we have not completely succeeded in this respect.
Lower left first molar	Indicates our desire to be loved by others. It quite often is the first one to be carious. This happens when the child tries to integrate its emotions and suffers emotional turmoil. The tooth is very painful when the child receives insufficient parental affection.
Lower right first molar	Stands for working life. It reflects difficulties one may have starting a company or working on projects. The tooth represents a new beginning, establishment or birth.

Teeth	Meaning
All second molars	They mirror the relationship we have to our surroundings. What image do we project onto our environment and what does it reflect on us?
Upper right second molar	Stands for external circumstances and our working life. A vigorous daredevil is more likely to have a healthy tooth, whereas an apathetic person or someone with escapist tendencies is likely to have a carious molar.
Upper left second molar	Indicates our emotional relationship to our fellows and to harmony between one another. In case someone is disappointed in a relationship, the tooth will develop problems.
Lower left second molar	It has a similar to the upper left second molar meaning. This means that disappointments in relationships have an even stronger impact on the condition of the tooth.

Teeth	Meaning
Lower right second molar	Stands for relationships and their circumstances. Constant quarreling may be responsible for damage to the tooth.
Wisdom teeth	They represent the energy that is connected with the collective and the individual consciousness. Furthermore they indicate our ability to align ourselves with the divine principle. Today it is quite common to systematically pull wisdom teeth. Thus, without wisdom teeth we are deprived easy access to the energy of the universe. It destroys the polarity that enables us to connect with the universal wisdom.

5. Glossary

Acne: Increased and pathologic secretion of sebum adenoids leads via increased hardening of the skin to the development of blackheads, nodules, pustules and sometimes scars.

Adaptation: Ability of organs to adapt

Allergy: The altered reaction of an organism based on antigen-antibodies following prior sensitization by antigens.

Amalgam: Mercury-metal-alloy

Bronchial asthma: Shortage of breath caused by cramping of the bronchia

Depression: Dispirited mood

Diabetes: Malfunction of the pancreas

Digestive enzyme: A bodily substance to accelerate digestion

Eczema: Most common itching, sporadically appearing, inflammable ailment of the epidermis and the papillae

Embryo: Fruit of the womb in the early stages of development, i.e. during the first three months of pregnancy

Endogenous depression: Physical depression without external trigger.

Furuncle(boil): Acutely purulent inflammation of a hair follicle and its sebum adenoid; painful, inflamed lump the size of a bean to a walnut with yellow middle point, a centered core of a boil surrounded by a severe edema.

Gastritis: Catarrh of the stomach, especially its mucous membrane, acute and chronic

Hormones: Active agents that are created in endocrine glands (glands with inner secretion) or in certain cells or tissues (tissue hormones). The hormones control metabolic processes in certain organs in a specific way.

Hypertension: High blood pressure, measured pressure exceeding 140/80 (160/80) of persons between 20 to 50 years of age

Immune system: Those structures of an organism that can be carriers of immune functions or where lymphatic cells develop or increase. These structures are primarily the lymphatic system.

Implant: A foreign part implanted in the body, in this case an artificial tooth

Lymphatic vessel: Vessel that returns lymph (a light yellow liquid consisting of lymphatic plasma and achroacytes) via lymph nodes (flat-round organs the size of a lentil to a hazelnut in the lymphatic system) to the blood circulation.

Meridians: In traditional Chinese medicine, channels on the surface of the body as well as within the body on which the acupuncture points are situated.

Oropharynx: Area of the throat behind the oral cavity leading to the ear

Oxidation process: Chemical process that adds oxygen to an element or a composition.

Pancreas: A digestive organ located behind the stomach

Pancreatitis: Inflammation of the pancreas

Periodontosis: Atrophy of the root of the tooth and surrounding tissue without inflammation, as a result of reduced vital energy of the tissue. Main symptom is loosening of the teeth.

Pituitary gland (hypophysis): Endocrine gland located at the base of the brain.

Psychosomatic medicine: Teaches the correlation of a physical ailment and its psychical cause.

Resection: Excision of a complete organ or diseased parts of it

Stress: State of increased activation of an organism

Temporary retainer (brace): Removable plastic cover for the teeth to correct the bite. The retainer brings the jaws into the right position and helps to reduce tooth grinding and pressing.

Tinnitus: Ear noises, buzzing or ringing in the ear, discernable by the patient but no one or nothing else. Tinnitus is not an ailment, but a symptom.

Toxins: Water-soluble poisonous substances from microbes, plants or animals having a certain incubation time, a specific effect and unknown chemical structure

Tumor: A diseased swelling in any part of the body

Vitality: Liveliness, physical strength and mental vigor

Vitamin deficiency: Deficiency of essential vitamins which can lead to impaired eyesight and rapid exhaustion of the eyes, dry mucous membranes, cracked lips, etc.

6. Recommended Reading

Adler, Dr. Ernesto: Störfeld und Herd im Trigeminusbereich, 5th edition, Heidelberg, Germany 2004

Berg, Dr. Dr. Stefan/Schmitz-Koep, Dr. Dr. Norbert: Schöne Zähne – Pflege, schmerzlose Behandlung, Zahnersatz, Implantate, Cologne, Germany

Caffin, Michele: Was Zähne zeigen, Braunschweig, Germany, 1997

Dahlke, R.: Krankheit als Symbol, Munic, Germany, 1996

Daunderer, Dr. Max: Amalgam, Sonderdruck, 6th edition, Landsberg/Lech, Germany, 2000

Gleditsch, Jochen M.: Reflexzonen und Somatotopien, Schorndorf, Germany, 1983

Gleditsch, Jochen M.: Mundakupunktur, Schorndorf, Germany, 1979

Graf, Dr.med.dent. Karlheinz: Ganzheitliche Zahnmedizin – Fakten, Wissenswertes, Zusammenhänge, Stuttgart, Germany, 2000

Grandjean, M./Bornhofen, P.: Warum denn so verbissen? Kiefergelenksstörungen – eine neue Volkskrankheit aus ganzheitlicher Sicht, 1st edition, Sulzberg, Germany, 2003

Greese, Dr.med. Dr.med.dent. Uwe: Jedes Kind kann gesunde Zähne haben – Der Kinderzahngesundheitsratgeber, 1st edition, Erlangen, Germany, 2003

Kares, Horst/Schindler, Hans/Schöttl, Rainer: Craniomandibuläre Dysfunktionen: der etwas andere Kopf- und Gesichtsschmerz, Hannover, Germany, 2003

Kiel-Hinrichsen, Monika/Kviske, Renate: Wackeln die Zähne, wackelt die Seele, 3rd edition, Stuttgart, Germany, 2004

Klein, Thomas: Energieverlust und Krankheit durch Zahnherde. Ein Wegweiser zur Selbsthilfe und Heilung, 1st edition, Dresden, Germany, 2004

Kramer, F.: Elektroakupunktur in der zahnärztlichen Praxis, Heidelberg, Germany, 1994

Kramer, F.: Lehrbuch der Elektroakupunktur, Heidelberg, Germany, 1976-1981

Maier, MR Dr.med. Reinhild: Gesunde Zähne ein Leben lang, 2nd edition, Leoben, Austria, 2002

Markert, Christopher: So retten Sie Ihre Zähne, 1st edition, Hopferau-Heimen, Germany, 1983

Mastalier, O.: Reflextherapien in der Zahn-, Mund- und Kieferheilkunde, Berlin, Germany, 1987

Mieg, Rosemarie: Zähne als Krankheitsursache, Munic, Germany, 1996

Mieg, Rosemarie: Krankheitsherd Zähne – Schnelle Heilung durch Erkenntnisse der Herdforschung, Bergisch-Gladbach, Germany, 1996

Müller-Fahlbusch, H.: Ärztliche Psychologie und Psychosomatik in der Zahnheilkunde, Stuttgart, Germany, 1992

Roissant, A./Lechner, J./Asche, R. van: Das cranio-sacrale System, Heidelberg, Germany, 1991

Roy, Ravi/Lage-Roy, Carola: Homöopathischer Ratgeber Zähne, 2nd edition, Murnau, Germany, 2001

Schneider, Dr. med. Elisabeth : Tinnitus & Tierkreiszeichen, 1st edition, Munic, Germany, 1999

Schreckenbach, Dr.med.dent. Dirk: An jedem Zahn hängt immer auch ein ganzer Mensch – Das Resümee eines Praktikers; die ganzheitliche Betrachtung und Verbindung von Körper, Geist und Seele bezogen auf den Mundraum und die Zähne, 4th edition, Homburg, Germany, 2004

Stiftung Warentest: Zähne Vorsorge Behandlung Kosten, 4th edition, 2005

Strittmatter, B.: Das Störfeld in Diagnostik und Therapie, Stuttgart, Germany, 1998

Tepperwein, K.: Die Botschaft deines Körpers, Triesen, Germany, 1984

Tepperwein, K.: Was dir deine Krankheit sagen will, Munic, Germany, 1990

Venanzi, Dr. Luigi/Spallone, Dr. Livio/Ferrarelli, Dr. Enrico: Die Aufbissschiene – Eine Platte zur Koordinierung der Kiefergelenksbewegung, 1st edition, Munic, Germany, 2004

Volkmer, Dietrich: Zähne natürlich gesund halten: sanfte Heilung durch biologische Zahnheilkunde, Munic, Germany, 1998

Voll, Reinhold: Wechselbeziehungen von Odontonen und Tonsilien zu Organen, Störfeldern und Gewebssystemen, 5th edition, Uelzen, Germany, 1996

Volz, Dr. Ulrich/Heinzel, Dr. Hauke/Lambrich, Dr. Martin/ Heidemann, Dr. Katrin/Maier, Joachim A. : Zähne gut – alles gut, Stuttgart, Germany, 2004

Personal Notes